Breathe Better

Health Advice
to
Improve Breathing

- Paul F. Davis -

Lifesaving and Life-Changing Book

- Health Advice

- Breathing Problems

- Respiratory Obstructions

- Nutritional Suggestions

- Increase Oxygen

- Environmental Health

- Vitamins and Mineral Supplements

Health Advice

Although I am not a medical doctor (thank God for that), I am a former lifeguard, personal fitness trainer, wellness trainer, and nutritional consultant. Remember medical doctors are trained in medical schools, which are heavily financed by pharmaceutical companies (their chief financiers which heavily lean on and influence medical schools to advocate a pill pushing paradigm that enriches drug companies rather than advocating and suggesting alternative medicine and holistic health remedies).

For legal purposes to cover my ass, like all others writing health books, I will tell you (although I myself don't believe it and certainly would never take this advice when seeking HEALTH); "ask your doctor" before doing anything. However you also may want to read "Dead Doctors Don't Lie"

(http://amzn.to/1q7BBGy) written by one brilliant medical doctor who compiled obituaries when doctors died and thereby proved doctors are not as smart as we think and error when caring for their own health. I know this to be true, because my grandmother's doctor smoked (and smoked so much it could be smelled on him, as his nurse confirmed with embarrassment when I asked).

The New York Times, Newsweek, and other reputable news sources have themselves written articles on the questionable ties of medical colleges with pharmaceutical companies (even to the extent of giving Harvard a D and near failing marks for ethics violations in taking pharmaceutical money and allowing it to influence the medical college students curriculum).

Furthermore many universities professors write in journals that are funded by pharmaceutical companies to achieve preordained conclusions (to favor the creation of a new drug, support the use of a drug, and increase the sales of a drug) to support the pharmaceutical industry and perpetuate their existence, not the furtherance of good health in humans as promised when physicians take a Hypocratic oath to obtain their medical license (because in the medical industry ongoing sickness is the money maker, not health). Thus the medical, psychiatric and pharmaceutical industries all thrive on creating new diseases, names for these diseases, keeping patients sick (but hopeful to improve) and thereafter creating new drugs to allegedly (though with multiple side affects) "cure" the problem (or dismantle the synergy and total wellness of the human body, by disrupting the body's immunity and connected inter-reliance to thereby ensure ongoing patient illness and sickness - thus making them a profitable patient for life).

Nevertheless since some will not believe me, I suggest reading a book written by a medical doctor and professor at Harvard Medical College on "How Doctors Think" (http://amzn.to/1k7ShMP), which acknowledges as reported by the American Journal of Medicine that doctors error in their diagnoses of patients up to 25% of the time.

Breathing Problems

I understand breathing problems personally because when I was born, I was put in an oxygen tent for the first month of my life, as I had pneumonia and nearly died. As the documentary film, "The Business of Being Born" reveals,

http://amzn.to/2eUk1DN

modern medicine is such that physicians and hospitals prey on patients to increase their profit margins (which sometimes involves unnecessary "interventions" to speed up the delivery, ease the doctor's workload, take the mother out of the picture via sedation, and thereafter let the doctor take control). Of course none of these approaches is good for the baby's health, nor the mother's (all the while severing the vitally important physical and emotional connection between the mother and baby).

In Africa, mothers give birth to their babies squatting and work with gravity so the baby drops and comes out nicely. One woman in Mozambique (in the middle of a treacherous storm) years ago, even gave birth in a tree. Thus giving birth without the assistance and nearby presence of medical doctors happens every day throughout Africa and many developing countries where I have traveled and lived.

The opposite occurs in the western world where the physician's comfort is the primary focus, which results in pregnant mothers being laid on their backs on an elevated table so doctors can easily access and deliver the baby. The only problem is natural child births sometimes can last many hours (as I discovered when my daughter was born under water in a Jacuzzi at a birth center with no doctors present - a beautiful and peaceful process that lasted 12 hours or more).

The midwife and doula were very kind, encouraging, patient and supportive. My wife laid in the warm Jacuzzi and mostly agonized right at the point of delivery, after which the joy of our daughter's birth filled us with incredible peace and emotional release.

I can only wish my own birth was as painless, glorious and free from medical intrusions and interference. Unfortunately, my mother was a smoker and likely slipped up a bit during her pregnancy, which quite possibly may have resulted in me nearly suffocating in the womb with pneumonia. Under this circumstance, the presence of medical doctors proved necessary and helpful (as I was put in an oxygen tent). Yet there is a possibility that my mother did not smoke during her pregnancy (as my father thinks she did not) and a medical intervention of some sort damaged my lung or lungs?

One thing is for certain, many pregnant young ladies who drink alcohol and smoke do not discover they are pregnant until a month or more into the pregnancy (all the while negatively impacting their baby's health with their consumption of alcohol and tobacco). Quite possible this can be much more fatal and deadly during the first month or two of pregnancy.

I cannot ask my mother today regarding this because she was killed by an 18 year old drunk driver. My father now has Alzheimer's and is getting up there in years.

Yet my studies of health and nutrition, as someone who has earned Master degrees in Health (University of Alabama) and Global Food Law (Michigan State College of Law) taught me about the problems with the American Medical Industry (an industry for profit, not truly motivated to serve people - as I personally have repeatedly experienced whenever I visited medical clinics, doctors offices, or hospitals in the United States and was asked for my social security number, credit card billing information, address, and to sign a stack of legal documents to ensure I paid for the visit; long before I ever saw or spoke to a doctor).

In fact often times the outdated medical drugs prescribed by doctors in the USA have horrible side effects resulting in death (such a Vioxx - a drug originally for treating arthritis created by Merck that killed over 500,000 people giving them heart attacks).

The devastating effect of Merck's drug Vioxx preying on the elderly (and exacerbating their arthritis as the body excretes calcium from the bones to remove such toxic drugs from the body) was evident throughout America because the year the toxic drug was introduced and went to market in 1999, this year showed the largest rise in the American death rate. Conversely, in 2004, when Vioxx was pulled from the drug market and kept from consumers, the death rate in America substantially declined. Thus Americans are often being killed by their pill pushing physicians for profit. Later studies by the United States Food and Drug Administration (FDA) proved that the use of Vioxx led to deaths from cardiovascular diseases such as heart attacks and strokes, reminding us all of the painful and deadly side effects of drugs (one claimed to solve one ailment, while causing several more, and in this case resulting in death).

https://www.legalexaminer.com/health/vioxx-killed-half-a-million-the-facts-are-grim/

https://www.theweek.co.uk/us/46535/when-half-million-americans-died-and-nobody-noticed

https://www.theamericanconservative.com/articles/chinese-melamine-and-american-vioxx-a-comparison/

It is therefore worth remembering that drugs are toxic, come with harmful side effects, and are often deadly (some "working" and delivering death more speedily than others). Therefore a holistic approach to health must be pursued by consumers and patients to avoid the deadly practices of physicians for profit seeking to prey on patients and monetize the moment.

Even antibiotics have now been eclipsed by morphing bacteria that now are becoming stronger and smarter than antibiotics. In fact most "super bugs" (viruses and infectious diseases) are now lingering and lurking in hospitals (as one pregnant mother in Orlando, Florida learned when giving birth to her baby; after which she was informed she picked up an infectious virus and must have her arms and legs amputated). So much for the days of happy child birth experiences at hospitals.

Medical interventions that speed up the delivery of babies have been scientifically researched extensively and said to increase the complications of the health of the baby at child birth; among the complications being respiratory problems. Giving mothers pain killers and epidurals can in fact hinder the well-being and health of the baby, by thwarting the natural delivery process, imparting toxic drugs into the mother (and thereby the baby connected at the umbilical cord) and hindering the baby's lung capacity and oxygen intake thereby.

Therefore it is vitally important to guard yourself from unnecessary medical interventions, which may profit the physician but not you the patient (nor your beloved children and family).

Removing a woman's uterus and ovaries is a questionable practice, as there are far better ways to deal with the underlying problem than to begin removing vital body parts and disrupting a woman's hormones. The same applies to removing a man's testicles (fearing testicular or prostate cancer) as testosterone in actuality helps heat up the body and kill cancer. Moreover testosterone gives men the ability to fight, the will to live and be a man (without which what man wants to remain alive).

Respiratory Obstructions

Having lived as a missionary and teacher in China, India, and Thailand (among other countries); I witnessed students habitually coughing (perhaps due to air pollution and also environmental pollution depending on where their parents live). The air we breathe, the water we drink and the food we eat greatly impacts our well being.

Chemical trails were continually being sprayed in the skies of Orlando, Florida (the last 10 years or more I lived there) directly over my home and neighborhood. Yet although my home was in the direct path of commercial airlines flying to and from MCO (airport); the chemical trails I am referring to (crisscrossing the sky overhead and destroying perfectly blue skies in the sunshine state of Florida) were in fact being sprayed by military and military contractor planes conducting environmental experimentation and geo-engineering across America (and many other NATO countries such as France - as I saw the same occur in Paris on a perfectly blue day overhead until a chem trail was sprayed in the sky).

Some allege these chem trails are intended to reduce the temperature in the sky and earth below to prevent global warming or climate change, others speculate they are for the intention of military practices to prepare our nation in the event of a war (so we have an additional advantage with such "technology" to be able to artificially manufacture weather patterns in our nation and others if the event of combat). Universities such as Carnegie Mellon and Harvard have commented on these practices online, the former even hosted an entire conference on the matter of geo-engineering.

Certainly ecocide occurred in Vietnam during the Vietnam War, when American planes sprayed "agent orange" overhead polluting the environment and soil below; resulting in four generations of babies being born with deformities (as I witnessed with my own eyes when traveling throughout Vietnam in 2011 and completing global intensive coursework there with New York University).

Here below are some videos I produced over the years on chemical trails polluting our skies overhead (without giving the citizens below a say or vote in the matter before our governments agree to and permit such experimentation to occur in the skies above us and directly affecting the health of us living below them).

Env Health Speaker, Respiratory Problems, Chemtrails Hybrid Parasite

https://www.youtube.com/watch?v=2svcAcCYhaM

Chemtrails Attorney - Chemtrails Lawyer - Chemtrail Health Violations

https://www.youtube.com/watch?v=Tq9N9rOb1IU

Chemtrail Parasites - Air Pollution - Trouble Breathing - Morgellons

https://www.youtube.com/watch?v=pacjai4A5XE

Env Experiments - Vietnam Ecocide - Birth Defects - Chemtrails

https://www.youtube.com/watch?v=8RmDj4mHde

M

Breathing Problems - Trouble Breathing - Chemtrails and Morgellons

https://www.youtube.com/watch?v=8NYX-

kYToXw

Ecocide - Vietnam War - Chemtrails - Public Health Speaker

https://www.youtube.com/watch?v=hYL767p1JfI

Chemtrails, NATO climate engineering, Morgellons parasite

https://www.youtube.com/watch?v=Pcj3nslbOmQ

Public Health Warning - Stop Chemtrails and Geo Engineering

https://www.youtube.com/watch?v=EX-Ih3MRsUA

Chemtrail Parasites - Air Pollution - Trouble Breathing - Morgellons

https://www.youtube.com/watch?v=pacjai4A5XE

Nerve Damage - Paralysis - Chemtrail Morgellon Parasite

https://www.youtube.com/watch?v=y5WrQIaDqQw

Medical doctor Hiromi Shinya, professor at Einstein Medical College in Manhattan, New York was embarrassed and humiliated when his beloved daughter had dermatitis and stomach problems, which he as a physician could not heal, correct, or resolve (as he states in his book "The Enzyme Factor" - http://amzn.to/192i6bM).

It was when this brilliant, resilient and persistent doctor created the colonoscopy to go inside and evaluate the stomachs of patients (he having been inside over 300,000 stomachs including those of celebrities and patients) that he realized meat and dairy are harmful to the gut, intestinal lining, cause inflammation and thus can at times hinder breathing and other bodily functions.

One of the best things to drink to remove parasites and rid the gut of candida and cancerous growths, I have personally found, is drinking aloe (which is more rich in oxygen than anything else you can eat or drink). My favorite aloe juice provider is Lily of the Dessert (from Arizona), which I typically would either buy online or at Whole Foods. I found online was cheaper here (and came in glass jars, which Whole Foods often did not have preferring plastic containers which I'm not a fan of as the plastics can leach into liquid substances).

Lily of the Desert Preservative Free Organic Inner Fillet Aloe Vera Juice, 128 Ounce - Supports Health Digestion

https://amzn.to/2J28ypM

Lily Of The Desert Juice Aloe Vera Pf Whl Lea

(32 ounces) - Glass Jar

https://amzn.to/2EOJUDK

Remember human beings can only live 2 minutes without oxygen. We can go 2 days without water and 40 days without food. Yet oxygen is so often neglected as the corporations of the world involved in heavy industry and manufacturing continue to use the skies above us as an open sewer (and thereby contaminate the air we all breathe and our water supply due to rainfall containing such hazardous and toxic chemicals from the skies).

My students habitually coughing would disrupt classes and themselves when trying to focus academically. It was then that I began making suggestions to them for helpful dietary supplements and natural remedies I myself take as a teacher living abroad in developing countries to strengthen my human immunity and prevent illness (as schools are common breeding grounds for viruses, bacteria and illnesses), much like prisons (where large groups of people congregate and interact closely).

Liver Cleanse to Detox

If you are overweight, have pain in your internal organs (like within your liver and gallbladder) being junked up and in need of a serious ongoing detox (both to lose weight and to improve your internal organs function and thereby your breathing); I recommend a liver cleanse (via coffee enemas) also called colonics by some who nurses and health clinics who administer this to help people repair, decontaminate and break free blockages within their digestive tract (wherein 60% or more of your immune system is found).

I will say this as a note of caution however, the first (and last - as I never did it again with the assistance of someone) colonics I did; afterward I think I slept for 12 hours (quite possibly because it drained my electrolytes and may have been excessive as colonics is done with a machine as opposed to a liver cleanse via a coffee enema or the olive oil and lemon juice combination (which I now do and prefer), the latter options both allow your body to determine naturally how much to remove via the anus - versus a machine with colonics just pulling stuff out of you at its own pace, and quite possibly as I experienced far too much).

I realize not everyone is keen to do such a thing, but if you understood how effective a properly performed liver cleanse is (as I felt 10 years younger and renewed within afterward); you would be less inclined to resist and more focused on the final outcome and improved results and health benefits.

In fact when I did coffee enemas, the first thing I would feel was my ears would open up (as when riding on a plane and ascending to higher altitudes). Although I do not fully understand it, I experientially know it to be true (every time I did a coffee enema - which I did for 2 years or more).

I experienced great results, an increase in energy and reduced internal burden on my body (which consistently comes through a polluted food and water supply, toxic environment in which we live, stress and so much more than we realize).

Cars get serviced and have oil and fluid changes. Yet human beings go through life never have any of these, which results in an automobile breaking down and ceasing to operate properly after about 10 years in service.

Hereafter I have created some videos to help you capture the essence of the liver, its vital functions, burdensome challenges, and ways to help detoxify your liver and body. These videos were made several years ago. I therefore apologize in advance for them, but not for the profound, enlightening and life-saving information therein. Should you want personalized attention, health coaching and wellness training; please contact me directly to schedule a paid consultation (RevivingNations@yahoo.com).

Detoxification - Liver Cleanse (1 of 2)

https://www.youtube.com/watch?v=hqMlZ0jPt1k

Detoxification - Liver Cleanse (2 of 2)

https://www.youtube.com/watch?v=34u_nBtgU74

Detox FDA Acetaminophen

Meds Drugs Liver Damage

https://www.youtube.com/watch?v=9hQq_L9FX0U

Coffee Cleanse - Coffee Enema (1 of 2)

https://www.youtube.com/watch?v=CdyrjGASHD
M

Coffee Cleanse - Coffee Enema (2 of 2)

https://www.youtube.com/watch?v=XLcjw8NHopc

Liver Cleanse - Fatty Liver (1 of 3)

https://www.youtube.com/watch?v=a4LqDQMNKv
k

Liver Cleanse - Improve Breathing (2 of 3)

https://www.youtube.com/watch?v=tzKfUVGZ0hE

Health Speaker - Liver Cleanse (3 of 3)

https://www.youtube.com/watch?v=kkNF57HLWA
w

Deadly Parasites - Parasite Cleanse

https://www.youtube.com/watch?v=untcwTVG_lo

**Health Coach, Wellness Speaker - Liver Cleanse
Steps (1of5)**

https://www.youtube.com/watch?v=9Vo1s2ZMGa
Q

**Health Coach, Wellness Speaker - Liver Cleanse
Steps (2of5)**

https://www.youtube.com/watch?v=sAQiNJCS1Rw
&t=1s

**Health Coach, Wellness Speaker - Liver Cleanse
Steps (3of5)**

https://www.youtube.com/watch?v=WsY83FkG_9
U

**Health Coach, Wellness Speaker - Liver Cleanse
Steps (4of5)**

https://www.youtube.com/watch?v=PBPyC7t4x-0

https://www.youtube.com/watch?v=YTacUg-5G2U

Nutritional Suggestions

Upon talking to an American nurse in China (at the school where I formerly taught) and a chemistry teacher, I discovered during a lunch conversation that raw honey is a natural antibiotic. It was that night when I went to the grocery store next door to my apartment to find the three darkest most pure appearing brand's of raw honey I could locate (from China, Europe and Australia) and began taking a teaspoon or a bit more daily; to strengthen my immunity. It truly worked because whenever I felt the slightest scratch in my throat or pain, after taking honey the mucus immediately came out of my throat and I began feeling better.

Dr. Hiromin Shinya is his book "The Enzyme Factor" (http://amzn.to/192i6bM) talks about papaya and pineapple having waste removing enzymes, which I highly recommend you eat regularly to help your body detox and heal itself.

Increase Oxygen

Also I recommend eating and drinking aloe juice (Lily of the Dessert is an excellent brand in the USA - https://amzn.to/2J28ypM) as aloe is rich in oxygen, which certainly helps increase your oxygen levels and remove cancer in the intestinal tract (where up to 60% of your immune system is found).

L-Arginine is an amino acid that increases nitric oxygen in the blood stream and energizes the body and male libido (https://amzn.to/2tZxe82). I highly recommend it and foods rich in L-Arginine.

Daily exercise (even if only walking) will improve your circulation, oxygen intake, and respiratory function. Whether you walk to work, outdoors for recreation, with your spouse after work, or to help the old lady across the street; all are good and beneficial (as is going to the local health club and burning fat via sweating on a stair master or treadmill).

Environmental Health

As the cancer villages of China have taught us, where soil is toxic from industrial dumping and disregard of heavy metals and toxic chemicals leaching into the soil and aquifer, consequently to pollute the rice grown therein; consumers of food need to be alert and aware as to WHERE their food comes from, HOW it is grown, WHO is growing it (and their values and motives - profit, sustainable profit, or a quality product to sustain generations with environmental ethics for the ecosystem and all complementary parts).

When Chinese in rural villages began getting sick, eventually they traced their illness to the poor environment in which the rice they were eating was grown. As a result, they stopped eating rice grown in a toxic and polluted environment, but continued to sell the same rich to unsuspecting consumers within the cities of their nation.

When we continually drink bad water, eat contaminated food, and breathe polluted air; these toxic inputs weaken our immunity and overall health. Medicine will not necessarily remove the toxic environmental inputs into our daily lives, but in fact will increase human toxicity.

Humans therefore must be alert and aware as to their environment and the impact of negative and toxic influences interfering with their well-being and disrupting the ecosystem and the humans living therein.

Ironically, many "air fresheners" and household "cleaning supplies" have toxic petro-chemicals within them that cause leukemia, cancer and many other illnesses in humans. The book "Solvent Neurotoxicity" - http://amzn.to/1hrlGNz (written by a PhD from Denmark) reveals how solvents used to mix various chemicals and concoctions are quite toxic - specifically benz, ethyl and benz.

Ten harmful solvents to take note of are: (Chloromethane; Dichloromethane; N-Hexane; Methyl Ethyl Ketone; Methyln N-Butyl Ketone; Styrene; Toluene; 1,1,1-Trichloroethane, Trichloroethylene, and Xylene) and two mixtures of solvents (White Spirit, Mixed solvent exposure) have been selected based on their widespread use, as well as the mounting evidence from research concerning the neurotoxicity of these particular solvents. Evidence from animal and human experiments, clinical observations, and epidemiological studies reveal their toxicity and how harmful they can be to human health.

Health conscious consumers, researchers, occupational hygiene specialists, epidemiologists, trade unions, construction and manufacturing department heads and foremen, along with industry leaders and employees working with organic solvents will find this book to be essential in determining methods for preventing chronic toxic neuropathy, encephalopathy, and other solvent-related disorders.

Just remember the only Benz you want in your life is a Mercedes (car). Otherwise get rid of the rest as benzene, removed from gasoline in the 1970s and reduced to a few parts per billion, causes leukemia and cancer. The U.S. Marine training base in Camp Lejeune found toxic benzene in their water supply, which caused families living on the military base to become very ill (some getting leukemia and cancer before dying and leaving us). The name of the documentary film exposing the incident is named "Semper Fi" (meaning always faithful) and can be seen at the web link hereafter: http://amzn.to/1Bvl2es

Solvent neurotoxicity causes acute and chronic neurotoxicity within humans via a number of harmful solvents commonly used in household cleaning supplies, cosmetics, air fresheners, and volatile chemicals even in car seats (to name just a few). These toxic chemicals can not only disrupt human hormones, but even make a car malfunction (as recently evidenced in the case of Sabaru when toxic perfumes and cleaning agents used therein made brake lights inoperable and defective).

The following articles below document in detail how toxic chemicals, particularly solvents, can impair automobiles and make manufacturing workers ill also.

https://www.caranddriver.com/news/a26595369/subaru-recall-impreza-forester-brake-lights/

https://www.ncbi.nlm.nih.gov/pubmed/27737812

https://www.tandfonline.com/doi/abs/10.1080/09638280110102126

https://www.ascentforums.com/forum/16-off-topic-discussion/6597-largest-subaru-recall-ever-brake-lights.html

The dirty dozen chemicals to watch out for are indeed ubiquitous and hard to avoid. These articles will serve as a further resource to perhaps guide you:

The Ugly Side of the Beauty Industry

https://amzn.to/2tWoz6p

Toxic Relief - Restore Health and Energy

https://amzn.to/2VPnwkF

Dirty Dozen 12 Ingredients to Avoid

http://ecodiscoveries.com/eco-friendly-green-cleaning-products-blog/dirty-dozen-12-ingredients-to-avoid-in-cosmetics-and-5-clean-beauty-brands-to-try/

Dirty Dozen Cosmetic Chemicals to Avoid

https://davidsuzuki.org/queen-of-green/dirty-dozen-cosmetic-chemicals-avoid/

Dirty Dozen 12 Toxic Chemicals in Makeup and Cosmetics You Must Avoid

http://www.alyaka.com/magazine/dirty-dozen-12-toxic-chemicals-makeup-cosmetics-must-avoid/

Vitamins and Mineral Supplements

Zinc is a powerful antioxidant and essential mineral vitally important for prenatal and postnatal development. Zinc deficiency negatively impacts up to two billion people around the world and is attributed to many diseases. Children with an insufficient supply of zinc in their bodies experience growth retardation, delayed sexual maturation, susceptibility to infection, and diarrhea.

I have experienced all of these in that I am not as tall as my father, did not reach puberty until I was 15 years of age, had allergies throughout my teenage years, often got sick when traveling overseas in developing countries, and had nonstop diarrhea in India for two months straight (and several other countries around the world when traveling as a missionary).

Zinc plating is used to reduce corrosion in iron and electrical batteries. Dietary supplements with zinc include zinc carbonate and zinc gluconate. Deodorants use zinc chloride. Anti-dandruff shampoos use zinc pyrithione to prevent dandruff. Excess zinc some believe causes copper deficiency, ataxia, and lethargy.

The world's zinc supply is largely deposited in Australia, Canada and the United States. The largest zinc reserves in the world however are in Iran. Zinc mines are mainly in China, Australia, and Peru.

Next to iron, aluminum, and copper; zinc is the fourth most commonly used metal in the world. Within dietary supplements, zinc comes in the following forms: zinc oxide, zinc acetate, zinc gluconate, and zinc picolinate.

Zinc deficiency has been associated with major depression. Zinc has been used extensively to treat children with diarrhea in the developing world (as the essential mineral is further depleted during diarrhea). Replenishing the body's zinc for two weeks and supplementing your daily allowance will lessen the likelihood of getting diarrhea or it reoccurring after already having it.

The good news is zinc picolinate (the form I use which is less hard on the stomach and more easily absorbed) is also excellent for improving the respiration of the lungs and thereby our ability to breathe without obstructions.

One study showed taking zinc supplementation reduces the progression of age related macular degeneration, which is to say zinc sustains and strengthens the eyes in humans.

Zinc also improves skin conditions such as dandruff and acrodermatitis enteropathica (a genetic disorder affecting zinc absorption that was fatal to infants). Intranasal sprays use zinc, but when used in excess can reduce a human's sense of smell.

The antimicrobial action of the ions in zinc improve the gastrointestinal tract and function, while also strengthening human immunity. Moreover large amounts of zinc when added to a urine sample, have the ability to mask the detection of drugs.

The inflammation within nasal passage way during the flu, common cold, and allergy season can be helped and mitigated by zinc. Thus many cold and flu remedies have zinc within them, especially throat lozenges.

My favorite form of zinc is NowFoods zinc picolinate in capsules for easy absorption accessible here: http://amzn.to/1WbrG3M

Taking beyond 75 milligrams a day within a 24 hour timeframe has been found to reduce cold and flu symptoms. By suppressing nasal inflammation, zinc has the ability to inhibit the human rhinovirus from replicating and spreading in the nasal mucosa within the nasal passageway.

Other forms of zinc that typically are less expensive (unlike the zinc picolinate, which I use from NowFoods) can result in nausea and a bad taste in one's mouth.

Topically, zinc oxide protects against sunburns in the summer and windburns in the winter. Likewise zinc oxide can prevent a baby from getting a diaper rash.

https://en.wikipedia.org/wiki/Zinc

More insightful articles with a wealth of information to help you on your journey to improve your breathing (and likely any skin ailments) are here after below.

Zinc and Respiratory Infections

https://www.who.int/elena/titles/zinc_pneumonia_children/en/

The Importance of Zinc in Respiratory Diseases

- https://www.asianscientist.com/2018/01/in-the-lab/lung-disease-zinc-cigarette-smoke/

New insights into the role of zinc in the respiratory epithelium.

https://www.ncbi.nlm.nih.gov/pubmed/11264713

Over the past 30 years, many researchers have demonstrated the critical role of zinc (Zn), in diverse physiological processes, such as growth and development, maintenance and priming of the immune system, and tissue repair. The physiology of zinc and its vital beneficial role in the respiratory epithelium is irrefutable. Zinc diversely acts as: (i) an anti-oxidant; (ii) an organelle stabilizer; (iii) an anti-apopototic agent; (iv) an important cofactor for DNA synthesis; (v) a vital component for wound healing; and (vi) an anti-inflammatory agent.

Thus zinc is a major dietary anti-oxidant, which has a protective role for the airway epithelium against oxy-radicals and other noxious agents. Zinc therefore has important implications for asthma and other inflammatory diseases where the physical barrier is vulnerable and compromised.

Once again here is the exact link to zinc picolinate to help improve your breathing and the health of your lungs:

http://amzn.to/1WbrG3M

The Great Windkeeper (direct link to buy online below) is another excellent and wonderful natural herbal supplement I learned about from Chinese acupuncture, which I have used with great results.

https://amzn.to/2IB5wZo

The "Great Windkeeper" seems to be some sort of herbal remedy with plum tea. My experience is it dries up the mucus and cause of inflammation with your gut and lungs. A couple days after I began to use "The Great Windkeeper" my bowel movement was a bit harder and compacted, as whatever was blocking my breathing from within my lungs and nose seemed to have dried up and came out the back end in the toilet like a brick.

Breathing better is truly worth it, as oxygen intake is vitally important for optimal and good health. Remember without oxygen, the human body cannot function and all energy and life within ceases to exist. Cardiopulmonary resuscitation requires ongoing oxygen flow to and through the lungs to strengthen and sustain the body.

Prayer for Health, Healing and Wellness

The Word of God is life (John 6:63) and also strengthens and energizes the body, the power of the resurrection in Jesus Christ by the Holy Spirit that raised Him from the dead will also bring life and health to your mortal body (Romans 8:11).

Therefore <u>please pray with me now out loud saying</u>:

"Dear Jesus, thank you for dying for me.
Come by the power of the Holy Spirit that rose You
from the dead and live big in me. Make my life and
health what it ought to be. Restore me physically,
mentally, emotionally, and spiritually to make me
whole. Heal me wonderful Jesus by your
supernatural power this very hour. Come blessed
Holy Spirit of the living God to comfort (John
14:26) and heal me in the midst of my bodily
ailments and weaknesses (Romans 8:26-27).
Remove my pain and suffering, causing me to
dwell, abide and live daily in divine health. Heal me
now in Jesus Name and impart newness of life to
me for which I shall give you all the glory. Thank
you dear God. Amen."

Upon praying this prayer if you felt the touch of God, supernatural fire (Luke 3:16), a quickening internally and/or physically; I'd love to hear from you.

Know assuredly God is for you and if He be for you nothing can stand against you (Romans 8). Know for sure, it is God's will in Christ Jesus to heal and deliver you so you can be well and whole (read Isaiah 53). Jesus did not only die for humanity's sins and iniquities on the cross, He also died for us to be healed physically and experience newness of life (Romans 6:4; 2Corinthians 5:17).

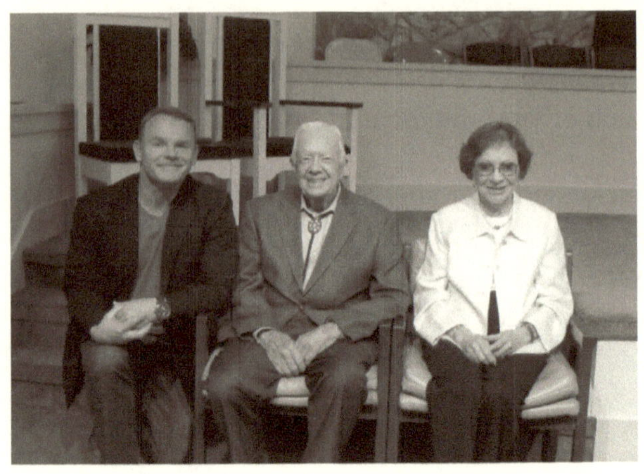

Paul with former United States President Jimmy Carter and his wife Rosalynn

Paul F. Davis is a University and Career Counselor who has worked at Texas A&M International University and for the American China Exchange Society. Paul has earned 4 Master degrees with the highest honors from the University of Texas (Educational Leadership), New York University (Global Affairs), Michigan State College of Law (Global Food Law), the University of Alabama (Health). Paul completed his training in University and Career Counseling at the University of California Los Angeles.

Paul is a Worldwide Motivational Speaker who has touched 89 nations speaking for the U.S. Military, Companies, Cruise Lines at Sea, Colleges and Universities throughout the globe.

Paul is the Author of 70+ books including:

- The Future of Food
- Geostrategy to Protect Environmental Health &
    Food Security
- Breakthrough For A Broken Heart
- Update Your Identity
- Integrity of Heart
- Educational Leadership and School Instructional
    Improvement
- College Admissions Secrets & Interview
    Strategies
- Charter Schools: Faith, Free Choice and Inferior
    Education for Profit Preying on Minorities
- United States of Arrogance
- Empowering & Liberating Women To Achieve
    Greatness
- Healthy Relationships
- Dating, Relationships, Love and Marriage

Many more books and videos can be seen at Paul's website below. Please also connect with Paul via social media.

www.PaulFDavis.com

www.EducationPro.us

www.Linkedin.com/in/worldproperties

www.Facebook.com/speakers4inspiration

www.Twitter.com/PaulFDavis

RevivingNations@yahoo.com

www.ingramcontent.com/pod-product-compliance
Lightning Source LLC
Chambersburg PA
CBHW051417250726

48655CB00003B/1094